Tailbone Pai

A Beginner's 3-Step Guide to Ma
Through Diet and Other Natural M
Recipes and a Meal Plan

Disclaimer

By reading this disclaimer, you are accepting the terms of the disclaimer in full. If you disagree with this disclaimer, please do not read the guide.

All of the content within this guide is provided for informational and educational purposes only, and should not be accepted as independent medical or other professional advice. The author is not a doctor, physician, nurse, mental health provider, or registered nutritionist/dietician. Therefore, using and reading this guide does not establish any form of a physician-patient relationship.

Always consult with a physician or another qualified health provider with any issues or questions you might have regarding any sort of medical condition. Do not ever disregard any qualified professional medical advice or delay seeking that advice because of anything you have read in this guide. The information in this guide is not intended to be any sort of medical advice and should not be used in lieu of any medical advice by a licensed and qualified medical professional.

The information in this guide has been compiled from a variety of known sources. However, the author cannot attest to or guarantee the accuracy of each source and thus should not be held liable for any errors or omissions.

You acknowledge that the publisher of this guide will not be held liable for any loss or damage of any kind incurred as a result of this guide or the reliance on any information provided within this guide. You acknowledge and agree that you assume all risk and responsibility for any action you undertake in response to the information in this guide.

Using this guide does not guarantee any particular result (e.g., weight loss or a cure). By reading this guide, you acknowledge that there are no guarantees to any specific outcome or results you can expect.

All product names, diet plans, or names used in this guide are for identification purposes only and are the property of their respective owners. The use of these names does not imply endorsement. All other trademarks cited herein are the property of their respective owners.

Where applicable, this guide is not intended to be a substitute for the original work of this diet plan and is, at most, a supplement to the original work for this diet plan and never a direct substitute. This guide is a personal expression of the facts of that diet plan.

Where applicable, persons shown in the cover images are stock photography models and the publisher has obtained the rights to use the images through license agreements with third-party stock image companies.

Introduction

If you are reading this, then chances are that you or someone you know is suffering from tailbone pain. Also known as coccydynia, this condition can be quite debilitating, making it hard to find relief.

Coccydynia is commonly caused by an injury to the coccyx, which is the bone at the very end of the spine. This can occur due to a fall, prolonged sitting, or childbirth. However, in some cases, the exact cause of tailbone pain is unknown.

While there are many treatments available for coccydynia, not all of them are effective. This can be frustrating for those who are dealing with this condition on a daily basis.

The good news is that there are natural methods that can help manage coccyx pain and improve your quality of life. This beginner's quick start guide will teach you everything you need to know about tailbone pain, including its causes, symptoms, and treatment options.

In this beginner's quick start guide, you will discover...

• What tailbone pain or coccydynia is about

• Symptoms and risk factors in tailbone pain

• Different ways to treat coccydynia

• Natural methods to manage the pain and discomfort of coccydynia

• Diet guide that helps in managing tailbone pain

What Is Tailbone Pain?

The tailbone pain, which is called coccydynia in the medical field, is a type of chronic pain that affects the coccyx, the other name for the tailbone. The coccyx is the bone at the very end of the spine and is located just above the buttocks.

On average, the human spine is made up of 33 vertebrae. These vertebrae are bones that protect the spinal cord and are divided into five sections:

• Cervical

• Thoracic

• Lumbar

• Sacral

• Coccygeal

The coccyx, located at the coccygeal, is the last bone in the spine and is made up of three to five fused vertebrae. It is a triangular-shaped bone that connects the sacrum—the name of the large bone at the base of the spine—to the pelvis, the bone that connects the legs to the trunk of the body.

The tailbone acts as a point of attachment for muscles and ligaments in the buttocks and lower back. It also helps absorb shock when we sit down or stand up.

Causes

It's common to think that coccydynia is usually caused by injuries, but even by doing mundane things, you may still experience pain in your tailbone. The usual causes of tailbone pain are as follows:

• Falling and landing on your buttocks

• Prolonged sitting

• Childbirth

However, in some cases, the exact cause of tailbone pain is unknown. There are several factors also that cause coccydynia, such as excessive weight gain, rapid weight loss, infection, tumor, and even aging.

The pain also ranges from a dull or mild ache to intense pain, or similar to a fierce stabbing pain. Cleveland Clinic categorized three different kinds of events that usually results in tailbone pain:

• **External Trauma**

This is when the coccyx becomes broken, bruised, or dislocated. This is usually caused by a fall or an accident, particularly when the buttocks and lower part of your body receive the most impact.

• **Internal Trauma**

This is when the coccyx pain is caused by trauma from sitting down on uncomfortable surfaces or positions for a prolonged period. This is because the coccyx is under constant pressure when we sit, which can irritate the bone and surrounding tissues. The reason why sitting is a common trigger for coccyx pain is because the coccyx is not meant to bear our body weight for long periods of time. This can cause the tissue around the coccyx to become inflamed, leading to pain and discomfort.

Difficult childbirth may also cause trauma to the tailbone. The act of pushing a baby out through the birth canal can put a strain on the coccyx, leading to coccydynia.

• Others

This is where other factors such as abscess, arthritis, infection, or tumor result in tailbone pain.

Despite these categorizations, however, it was learned that for about a third of those with coccydynia, the cause for their condition is usually undetermined.

Recognizing Tailbone Pain

Symptoms

The most common symptom of coccydynia is pain in the coccyx. This pain can range from mild to severe and may be sharp or dull. It may get worse when sitting, standing, or during certain activities.

Other symptoms of coccydynia include pain when moving the bowels, pain during sexual intercourse, and numbness or tingling in the buttocks.

Risk Factors

In particular, women are five times more likely to develop coccydynia than men. Anatomically, a woman's tailbone is positioned in a less-protected location compared to a man's. Women are also prone to get tailbone injuries due to pregnancy and childbirth.

However, this does not mean men don't experience tailbone pain as well. Just as previously mentioned, there are several risk factors that can increase your chances of developing coccydynia. These include the following:

• Aging: The risk of coccydynia increases with age. This is because the coccyx can become more fragile and susceptible to injury as we age.

• Being overweight: Excess weight puts extra pressure on the coccyx, which can lead to pain and discomfort.

• Rapid weight loss: Extreme and rapid weight loss may result in losing the padding protecting the coccyx, which may make it more vulnerable to injuries.

• Prolonged sitting down: Sitting down on a hard surface or on a narrow space can put a strain on the coccyx and lead to internal trauma to it.

• Previous injury to the tailbone: Previous injuries to the tailbone can make it more likely to develop coccydynia. Repetitive Strain Injury (RSI) happens when a person is engaged in a repetitive activity such as sports like cycling and rowing. These sports require the athlete to stretch the spine by leaning back and forth. Repetitive activities like that can strain the tissues around your coccyx.

Diagnosis

Coccydynia is typically diagnosed based on a medical history and physical examination. Your doctor will ask about your symptoms and any potential injuries or other health conditions that may be causing your pain. Your doctor may also look out for signs of an infection, arthritis, or other conditions that could be causing your pain.

For example, if you have pain in other areas of your spine, you may have a herniated disc or spinal stenosis. In some cases, imaging tests, such as X-rays, MRI, or CT scans, may be ordered to rule out other causes of coccyx pain or to assess the severity of the condition.

An MRI is a medical imaging procedure that allows doctors to look at the internal structures of the body without making any incisions. MRI machines use magnetic fields and radio waves to create detailed images of the inside of the body. MRIs are very useful for diagnosing problems with the brain, spine, and other soft tissues.

A CT scan is a medical imaging procedure that uses x-rays to create detailed images of the inside of the body. CT scans are very useful for diagnosing problems with the brain, spine, and other soft tissues.

Treating Tailbone Pain

There are various ways to treat and manage tailbone pain. There are available medications and home remedies that you can do when the pain becomes unbearable. It may be helpful to remember though that the pain rarely lasts for a lifetime.

Nonsurgical treatments

There are different types of treatments doctors will require depending on the severity of the coccydynia or tailbone pain. Here are the first two that may initially be recommended:

• **Physiotherapy** – this treatment aims to manipulate the muscles surrounding the coccyx in an attempt to ease the pain. Doing this may help in getting the coccyx to align better, which results in relief when urinating or defecating. Also part of the therapy is using cushions that make sitting down more comfortable.

• **Coccygeal injections** – these injections include a numbing agent or local anesthesia and a corticosteroid or a steroid that helps reduce inflammation.

Relief after injections is usually felt after 2 to 7 days. Then, depending on the person and the severity of the tailbone pain, the injections' effects may last for days, months, or even years. Ideally, stretching exercises are encouraged to be done during recovery. The doctor may also recommend another schedule for the injections, but take note that it shouldn't be done more than 3 times a year.

Surgical treatments

In case these two treatments aren't enough to lessen the pain and discomfort caused by the tailbone pain, surgical options are also recommended by doctors, but both are done very rarely. Usually, when the tailbone pain becomes unbearable, doctors would recommend nonsurgical treatments for at least a couple of months to about eight months before surgery is considered.

• Partial coccygectomy – only part of the coccyx is removed. While this is extremely rare, it's known to have a low complication rate and is considered an effective treatment.

• Total coccygectomy – entire coccyx or tailbone is removed. Similar to partial coccygectomy, it also has a low complication rate and is considered an effective treatment but is rarely done.

Both types of surgeries require a long recovery time, which may take a few months to about a year. It's also fairly uncomfortable, thus it is rarely recommended.

Natural Methods to Manage Tailbone Pain

There are people who are able to deal with the pain without receiving medications and home remedies. Usually, these are cases where the condition doesn't fully affect the quality of life of the patients. However, for those who do, there are different ways they can do to manage the pain and discomfort. One of the most common is taking NSAID (nonsteroidal anti-inflammatory drug) ibuprofen for the pain and swelling. Just make sure that you get or follow the prescribed number of ibuprofen to take for a period of time by your doctor.

Some of the most basic home remedies you can try to manage the pain are as follows:

Apply ice and heat

Applying ice to the area can help reduce swelling and pain. Heat can also help reduce pain and stiffness in the coccyx area. Heat increases blood flow to the area, which helps to reduce pain. Remember that either should be applied for no more than 20-30 minutes at a time.

Take vitamins and supplements

Usually, tailbone pain is associated with deficiencies in vitamins B6, B12, and D. It is known that a lack of these vitamins in one's diet may lead to painful bone inflammation. Thus, it's fairly normal for your doctor to recommend you take vitamins and supplements to help manage your condition and help nourish your bones.

There are a number of vitamins and supplements that can help reduce coccyx pain. Vitamin C is an antioxidant that helps to reduce inflammation. Vitamin B12 is important for nerve function and can help to reduce nerve pain. Vitamin D is great for calcium and phosphorus absorption, as well as for promoting the normal immune system.

Improving posture when sitting

One of the best things you can do for tailbone pain is to keep your spine in alignment. This means sitting up straight and avoiding slouching.

One of the reasons why slouching is so bad for tailbone pain is because it puts extra pressure on the coccyx. When you slouch, your spine is not in its natural position, and this can lead to pain and discomfort.

Another reason why posture is so important is that it helps to keep your muscles and joints in alignment. This alignment allows your muscles and joints to work together more efficiently, which can help to reduce pain and improve function.

There are a few things you can do to improve your posture when sitting:

• Sit up straight in a chair with your feet flat on the floor.

• Keep your knees at a 90-degree angle.

• Avoid crossing your legs.

- Lean forward when sitting down, keeping your back straight.

- Try not to sit for an extended period. Take breaks often to move around and stretch.

- Use lumbar support if you need to. Lumbar supports are devices that you can place in the small of your back to improve your posture and reduce pressure on your spine.

There are certain supportive pillows for the tailbone which are available on the market. For example, U-shaped pillows and doughnut-shaped pillows are designed to reduce pressure on the coccyx.

Refrain from sitting too long

If possible, try to avoid sitting for long periods of time as this can irritate the coccyx. If you must sit, take care to follow the recommended tips when sitting down listed above.

The reason why sitting can be so painful is that it puts pressure on the coccyx. This can happen when you sit in any chair, but it's more likely to happen if you sit in a hard chair or on a surface that isn't padded.

If you must sit, remember that it's best to take breaks every 20 to 30 minutes and to get up and move around for a few minutes. This will help keep your blood flowing and reduce the pressure on your tailbone.

Do some stretching and strengthening exercises

Simple coccyx-friendly exercises can help to improve the function of the muscles and joints around it. These exercises can also help to reduce pain and discomfort.

There are a few different stretching and strengthening exercises that you can do. The exercises listed below are great for stretching and strengthening the muscles around the coccyx.

Pelvic tilts: Lie on your back with your knees bent and your feet flat on the floor. Tilt your pelvis towards your chest, hold for a few seconds, and then return to the starting position. Repeat this exercise 10 times.

Clamshells: Lie on your side with your knees bent and your feet together. Lift your top knee up towards your chest, hold for a few seconds, and then return to the starting position. Repeat this exercise 10 times.

Hip abductions: Lie on your side with your knees bent and your feet together. Lift your top leg up in the air, hold for a few seconds, and then return to the starting position. Repeat this exercise 10 times.

There are many other stretching and strengthening exercises that you can do to help reduce pain and improve function. If you are unsure of how to do these exercises, you can ask your doctor or physical therapist for help.

Here are other tips you can follow to help improve the quality of your life and somehow alleviate the pain:

• Use a coccygeal cushion when sitting.

• To help with bowel movements, take stool softeners.

• When your lower back muscles are tense and in pain, take a hot/warm bath with Epsom salt.

• Avoid wearing tight-fitting clothes.

Tailbone pain can be a debilitating condition, but there are many things you can do to reduce pain and improve function. By following these tips, you can help to reduce your tailbone pain and live a more comfortable life.

Managing Tailbone Pain through Diet

A healthy and nutritious diet is always a good idea, even when your problem is the pain you're experiencing in your tailbone. Actually, when you consume food that's easy to digest, you're relieving yourself of the tailbone pain you may experience.

Constipation could also be a cause of discomfort and pain on your tailbone. When you are constipated, you put unnecessary strain on your tailbone when you poop. This can lead to pain and inflammation. To avoid these, here are some of the things you can do or change with your diet that will be great in managing tailbone pain.

Consume a high fiber diet

Eating a high-fiber diet is one of the best ways to prevent and treat constipation. Fiber adds bulk to your stool and helps it move through your digestive system more easily.

The recommended amount of fiber is 25 grams per day for women and 38 grams per day for men. Good sources of fiber include fruits, vegetables, whole grains, beans, and nuts.

You should also make sure to drink plenty of fluids. Water is the best choice, but you can also get fiber from fruit juices and other beverages. Soups are also a great source of fluids, especially those cooked with high-fiber ingredients.

Take fiber-rich supplements

If you are struggling to get enough fiber from your diet, you can also take a supplement. Psyllium husk is a type of soluble fiber that is often used as a supplement. It comes in powder form and can be added to water or juice.

Laxatives are another option, but they should only be used as a last resort. You may also want to consider taking a milder type of laxatives, also called stool softeners. Take note though, that some laxatives can make constipation worse if they are used too frequently.

Foods to Eat

Here are some foods that can help you prevent and treat constipation:

Whole grains

- barley

- brown rice

- oats

- whole wheat bread

Fruits and vegetables

- apples

- broccoli

- Brussels sprouts

- cabbage

- oranges

- pears

- prunes

Beans and legumes

- black beans

- kidney beans

- lentils

Nuts and seeds

- almond

- chia seed

- flaxseed

As mentioned in the earlier chapters, consuming fluids is highly recommended to help with your digestion. Aim to drink 8-10 glasses of water, including other liquids like juice or tea, per day.

As it was stated above, adding fiber to your diet will be very beneficial for you. However, here's something you need to remember. There are some people who have a hard time digesting fiber-rich food, and consuming more of it usually results in constipation. If you are one of those people, make sure that you consult with your doctor on how to modify your diet so you won't have to deal with constipation.

Foods to Avoid

There are some foods that can make constipation worse. These include:

Processed foods – Foods that are high in refined carbohydrates, such as white bread and pasta, can contribute to constipation.

Dairy products – Milk, cheese, and other dairy products can sometimes make constipation worse. If this is the case for you, try switching to a dairy-free diet or limiting your intake of dairy products.

Red meat – Eating too much red meat can lead to constipation. If you eat meat, make sure to choose leaner cuts of meat and balance it with other sources of protein, such as chicken or fish.

Caffeine – Caffeine can dehydrate your body and make constipation worse. If you drink caffeinated beverages, make sure to also drink plenty of water.

Alcohol – Alcohol can also dehydrate your body and make constipation worse. If you drink alcohol, make sure to also drink plenty of water.

7-Day Meal Plan

To help you get started with doing a non-constipation diet, let's start by making a meal plan that's perfect for a week. Making meal plans ahead of time is a great way to help you prepare ingredients and recipes that include food items highly recommended for you to consume. You can also plan ahead your grocery list so you can have a stress-free shopping spree, especially if you want to make sure to avoid stocking up on junk food.

Below is a sample 7-day meal with recipes included in this guide. This guide can be modified according to your preference.

	Breakfast	**Lunch**	**Dinner**
Day 1	Blueberry Pancakes	Aubergine Teriyaki Bowls	Crock Pot Chicken Soup
Day 2	Spinach Quiche	Pecan and Maple Salmon	Shrimp Avocado Salad
Day 3	Apple Cinnamon Smash Oatmeal	Sun Crust Turkey Cuts	Salmon Soup
Day 4	Cherry-Coconut Porridge	Avocado and Salmon Salad	Barley and Chicken Soup
Day 5	Veggie Omelet	Tuna Salad	Baked Turkey Wings
Day 6	Macrobiotic Apple and Oats Porridge	Tomato and Turkey Panini	Salmon and Fennel Salad
Day 7	Keto Zucchini Walnut Bread	Tuna and Veggies Wrap	Apple and Onion Soup

A 3-Step Plan Implementation

Now that you have learned a few methods to naturally treat tailbone pain, here is a 3-step plan to get you started:

Step 1 – Talk to your doctor

There are different ways to naturally manage tailbone pain, and most of them can actually be done at home. However, it's always still best to consult with your doctor first before trying or following these methods. This way, you can be assured that what you're doing is right, and you'll also be able to understand how exactly these methods help you.

For example, one of the most common suggestions to help manage or at least avoid tailbone pain is by modifying your diet by adding more fiber to it. However, because some people actually experience constipation when they consume more fiber, doing so without knowing if you're one of those people or not will definitely not be helpful for you. This is why it's important to talk to your doctor before going on a diet even if your goal is more about managing the discomfort you feel in your coccyx and not exactly losing weight.

It's also important that you talk to your doctor about vitamins and supplements you can take that will be helpful and not harmful to you. Even the more seemingly harmless things such as hot or cold compress, warm baths, compression cushions, and posture-correcting tools, make sure that you ask for your recommendations as well.

Remember that consulting with your doctor doesn't only happen before you start doing these things. You should regularly see your doctor so they could help you see if what you've done actually helped you or not. This way, you can also tweak the things you've done and make them more apt to your lifestyle.

Step 2 – Stick to a healthy diet and keep a food diary

As you start following a stricter diet that will be very helpful to your bowel movement, try to keep a food diary where you'll take note of how each meal made you feel. While it may seem tedious at first, you'll find that doing so will be beneficial for you in the long run.

You should be able to keep watch of the food that is easier to digest. You can also keep an eye on when you have trouble digesting or with your bowel movements.

Starting a diet is always stressful and challenging because it enforces you to change not only your usual menu but also your eating habits. Keeping a diary where you can write down your struggles or keep notes of your ups and downs during the diet journey can somehow lessen the burden of these major changes.

Step 3 – Stay consistent

While tailbone pain can be debilitating, especially when it's acting up, it doesn't mean you should just endure the pain and live with it. Try to do the routines that help you manage or alleviate the pain when you can. If the pain is unbearable, do the hot/cold compress or have a warm bath. If you can move a little, do the stretching and strengthening exercises. While these may not exactly cure your tailbone injury, they may help you feel more comfortable and make your day more bearable.

It also helps if you stay consistent in doing other little things that help you in the long run. For example, wearing loose-fitting clothes may not seem much, but if you somehow feel much more comfortable doing so, then do it.

Another thing that you must be consistent with is correcting your posture, whether you're standing up or sitting down. Again, this may not seem much, but once you become aware of it and do it more frequently, you'll definitely notice the difference compared to when you weren't correcting your posture. Doing so will help with aligning your bones and lessening the pressure on your tailbone, especially when you're sitting down. Use cushions and other posture-correcting tools to help with this if necessary.

After a long day, rest and do after-care. When you feel the pain in your tailbone becoming unbearable, apply either a hot or a cold compress, whichever you prefer that helps you feel better or what your doctor recommended. You can also do an Epsom salt bath to help you relieve the discomfort and pain.

We all know that consistency is key, so why not manage to make an effort to stick to the things that help you feel better and consistently do them? This 3-step plan may seem too simple, but actually, trying and implementing each step could actually greatly benefit you in the long run.

Sample Recipes

Blueberry Pancakes

Ingredients:

- 3 omega-3 fresh eggs
- 1 tsp. cinnamon
- 1/2 cup of arrowroot powder
- 1/4 cup of coconut oil
- 1/4 cup walnuts, roughly chopped
- 1 pinch sea salt
- 1/2 tsp. baking soda
- 1/2 tsp. yeast
- 1/2 cup coconut flour
- 1 tsp. vanilla extract
- 1/2 tbsp. lemon juice
- 1-pint blueberries

Instructions:

1. Whisk 3 eggs. Pour vanilla, lemon juice, and almond milk. Mix well.

2. In another bowl, combine arrowroot, salt, yeast, baking powder, cinnamon, and coconut flour. Add wet mixture to this mixture while whisking continuously.

3. Fold in the chopped walnuts.

4. Grease a saucepan over medium heat with coconut oil.

5. Once the oil is hot, scoop the mixture with a ladle, and pour the pancakes into the saucepan. Cook until bubbles form. Repeat this step until the batter is consumed.

6. For the sauce, simmer blueberries in another saucepan.

7. Add 4 tsp. of water. Simmer for 10 minutes.

8. Pour the sauce over a stack of pancakes and serve.

Apple Cinnamon Smash Oatmeal

Ingredients:

- 1-1/2 cups plain almond milk

- 1 cup oats

- 1 large Granny Smith apple

- 1/4 tsp. ground cinnamon

- 2 tbsp. toasted walnut pieces

Instructions:

1. Heat apple and oats together on a low to medium fire for about 5 minutes.

2. Add cinnamon.

3. Serve hot.

Spinach Quiche

Ingredients:

- 1 lb. breakfast sausage

- 1/2 onion, diced

- 2 cups mushrooms, sliced

- 6 cups spinach, roughly chopped

- 12 eggs

- 1/4 to 1/2 cup full-fat coconut milk

- 1 tsp. garlic powder

- 1 tsp. Italian seasoning

- 1 tsp. salt

- 1 tsp. pepper

Instructions:

1. Preheat the oven to 400°F.

2. Heat a cast-iron pan or another oven-safe pan over medium heat.

3. Cook sausage and onion. Stir occasionally until sausage turns brown, about 7-8 minutes.

4. Add in mushrooms. Allow them to cook with the sausage until soft, for about 2 minutes. Remove from heat.

5. Crack eggs into a large bowl.

6. Add coconut milk. For a lighter and fluffier texture, use ½ cup. Use less for less coconut taste.

7. Whisk together well to get a light egg mixture.

8. Add spinach and seasonings to the bowl with the eggs.

9. Add the sausage mixture to the bowl with the rest of the ingredients.

10. Mix until everything is well blended.

11. Line the pan with some fat from the sausage or grease well with oil, butter, or ghee to prevent quiche from sticking.

12. Pour mixture into the cast iron pan or oven-safe dish.

13. Bake for 40-45 minutes or until a knife poked at the center comes out clean.

14. Serve and enjoy while warm.

Cherry-Coconut Porridge

Ingredients:

- fresh or frozen cherries

- 1-1/2 cups oats

- 4 tbsp. of chia seeds

- 3 tbsp. of raw cacao

- 3-4 cups coconut milk

- a pinch of stevia

- coconut shavings

- dark chocolate shavings

- maple syrup

Instructions:

1. Combine oats, cacao, Stevia, and coconut milk in a small saucepan.

2. Boil over medium heat. Simmer until the oats are well-cooked.

3. Pour into a bowl. Top with cherries, coconut shavings, maple syrup, and dark chocolate shavings.

Veggie Omelet

Ingredients:

- 4 tsp. extra-virgin olive oil
- 1 small onion, finely chopped
- 4 pieces plum tomatoes, finely chopped
- 10 oz. spinach, chopped
- salt, to taste
- freshly ground black pepper, to taste
- 12 pcs. of egg whites
- 2 tbsp. water
- non-stick cooking spray

Instructions:

1. Cook onions, tomatoes, and spinach on a small skillet over medium heat. Add a pinch of salt.

2. Cook for about 3 to 5 minutes, or until the onion is soft.

3. Add pepper and another pinch of salt. Cook for another minute.

4. Remove the spinach and add it to a bowl. Cover and keep warm.

5. In a separate bowl, whisk egg whites and add water and a pinch of salt and pepper. Keep whisking until frothy.

6. Heat the skillet coated with cooking spray over medium heat.

7. Pour over 1/4 of the egg whites. Swirl all over the pan to evenly cover it. Cook for about a minute or two.

8. Lift the egg and allow the runny parts to flow underneath.

9. Spread about 1/4 tablespoon of the spinach into the omelet. Fold over the other side of the egg.

10. Once firm, slide the cooked omelet onto a serving plate.

11. Repeat with the remaining spinach and egg whites.

12. Serve.

Keto Zucchini Walnut Bread

Ingredients:

- 3 large eggs
- 1/2 cup virgin olive oil
- 1 tsp. vanilla extract
- 2-1/4 cups fine almond flour
- 1-1/2 cups sweetener, erythritol
- 1/2 tsp. salt
- 1-1/2 tsp. baking powder
- 1/2 tsp. nutmeg, ground
- 1 tsp. cinnamon, ground
- 1/4 tsp. ginger, ground
- 1 cup zucchini, grated
- 1/2 cup walnuts, chopped

Instructions:

1. Preheat your oven to 350°F.

2. Whisk together the eggs, oil, and vanilla extract. Set aside.

3. Using another bowl, combine the baking powder, sweetener, almond flour, salt, cinnamon, nutmeg, and ginger powder. Set aside.

4. Squeeze the excess water from the zucchini using a paper towel or a cheesecloth.

5. Pour the zucchini into the egg mixture and whisk.

6. Add the flour mixture slowly into the egg and zucchini mixture. Blend using an electric blender until the mixture turns smooth.

7. Spray a loaf pan with avocado oil or baking spray.

8. Pour the zucchini batter into the loaf pan and smoothen the top evenly.

9. Spoon the chopped walnuts on top of the batter, lightly pressing the walnuts with the back of a spoon to press into the batter.

10. Pop the loaf pan into the oven and then bake for 60-70 minutes, or until the walnuts turn brown.

11. Cool in a cooling rack before slicing and serving.

<u>Macrobiotic Apple and Oats Porridge</u>

Ingredients:

- 1 cup oats

- water

- 5 cups apples, cubed

- Stevia sweetener, to taste

- cardamom

- juice from 1 pc lemon

- raisins, for toppings

Instructions:

1. Cook oats in a small pan until done.

2. Add the ingredients and mix to combine on medium to low heat.

3. As the apples soften, take off the heat.

4. Serve with raisins on top of the oats.

Aubergine Teriyaki Bowls

Ingredients:

- 120 g jasmine rice

- 1 pc. aubergine, cut into large pieces

- 1-1/2 tbsp. vegetable oil

- 1 carrot, shredded

- 2 pcs. spring onions

- 1 clove garlic, crushed

- 1 ginger, finely grated

- 2 tbsp. soy sauce

- 1 tbsp. caster sugar

- 75 g frozen edamame beans

- a handful of radish, thinly sliced

- 1 lime, half juiced, half sliced

- 2 tbsp. toasted sesame seeds

Instructions:

1. Place rice into a pan with 240 ml. of water and a pinch of salt.

2. Boil and cook for a minute before simmering down to low heat for 10 minutes.

3. Let it steam for 10 minutes.

4. Put aubergine in the bowl and add 1 tbsp. oil.

5. Cook aubergine well.

6. Tip carrots, onions, ginger, and garlic, and then stir-fry until they become soft.

7. Whisk together soy sauce, sugar, and water. Pour it in.

8. Simmer down for 10 minutes until the aubergine becomes very soft.

9. Boil the frozen edamame beans. Drain and rinse in cold water.

10. Place them into a bowl with radish, seasoning, and lime. Toss well.

11. Place rice into the bowls.

12. Top it with aubergine, sauce, and other ingredients.

Avocado and Salmon Salad

Ingredients:

- 1/4 avocado, peeled with pit discarded

- 1 tbsp. lemon juice

- 2 tsp. extra-virgin olive oil

- 1 tsp. Dijon mustard

- salt

- freshly ground black pepper

- 4 oz. canned wild salmon, with bones, no salt added

- 2 tbsp. celery, sliced

- 2 tbsp. parsley, finely chopped

Instructions

1. In a medium bowl, combine the avocado, lemon juice, olive oil, mustard, salt, and pepper.

2. Mash the avocado with the back of a fork, and combine thoroughly with the other ingredients.

3. Flake the salmon, and add it to the avocado mixture.

4. Add the celery and parsley.

5. Serve immediately.

Tuna Salad

Ingredients:

- 1/2 cup pecans

- 1 cup chicken breast, steamed and cubed

- 1 cup tuna in oil

- salt, to taste

- pepper, to taste

Instructions:

1. Mix all ingredients in a large bowl.

2. Add a dash of salt and pepper to taste.

3. Chill for at least an hour before serving.

Salmon and Fennel Salad

Ingredients:

- 4 pcs. skinless salmon filets
- 2 tsp. parsley, chopped finely
- 1 tsp. thyme, chopped finely
- 2 tbsp. olive oil
- 4 cups fennel, sliced
- 1 clove garlic clove, grated
- 2 tbsp. orange juice
- 1 tsp. lemon juice
- 2/3 cup greek yogurt
- 2 tbsp. dill, chopped

Instructions:

1. Preheat the oven to 200°F.

2. Take a small bowl, and add the thyme and parsley. Stir them well.

3. Put the salmon over a flat surface and brush some oil. Sprinkle the mixed herb mixture evenly.

4. Place 2 filets at a time in the air fryer basket. Cook them for 10 minutes at 350°F.

5. Once done, transfer them to the preheated oven to keep warm. Repeat the process with the remaining salmon filets.

6. In a medium-sized bowl, add the sliced fennel along with grated garlic, yogurt, dill, lemon juice, orange juice, and remaining salt. Toss them well.

7. Serve the filets hot over the fennel salad.

Pecan and Maple Salmon

Ingredients:

- 4 pcs. of 4 oz. salmon fillet

- 1/2 tsp. onion powder

- 1/2 tsp. chipotle pepper powder

- 1 tbsp. apple cider vinegar

- 1 tsp. smoked paprika

- 1/2 cup pecans

- salt

- ground black pepper

- 3 tbsp. pure maple syrup

Instructions:

1. Lay salmon fillets on a baking sheet.

2. Season them with salt and pepper.

3. In a food processor, pulse in pecans, vinegar, maple syrup, chipotle powder, paprika, and onion powder in a food processor. Continue doing so until the texture becomes crumbly.

4. Coat the top of the salmon fillet with the pecan mixture.

5. Place the fillet in the refrigerator without cover for about 2-3 hours.

6. Preheat the oven to 425°F.

7. Bake the salmon fillet for about 12-14 minutes, or until the fillet flakes easily with a fork.

Shrimp Avocado Salad

Ingredients:

Salad:

- 1/2 lb. large shrimp, peeled
- 2 sweet corn ears, removed from the cob
- 4 cups Romaine lettuce, chopped
- 3 strips of bacon, diced
- 1 avocado, peeled, pitted and diced
- Optional: 1/3 cup Fontina cheese, grated

Buttermilk pesto dressing:

- 1/2 cup buttermilk
- 1/4 cup pesto, homemade or store-bought
- 1/2 cup mayo or Greek yogurt
- 1 tbsp. lemon juice
- 1 small shallot, minced
- salt
- pepper

Instructions:

1. Over high heat, place a skillet.

2. Put in the corn kernels when the skillet heats up.

3. Allow to dry roast while stirring occasionally. Cook until the edges start to caramelize and turn brown, or for about 6-8 minutes.

4. Place the roasted corn on a plate and set aside.

5. Lower the heat to medium-high. Fry the bacon using the same skillet, for about 6 minutes, until crispy.

6. Transfer the bacon to a plate.

7. Saute the shrimp in the same skillet until they are cooked.

8. In a bowl, toss the lettuce, corn, avocado, bacon, and shrimp.

9. Whisk all the ingredients together until blended.

10. Season with salt and pepper.

Tuna and Veggies Wrap

Ingredients:

- 1 canned tuna

- 2 pcs. whole-grain tortillas

- 1 cup cucumber, sliced

- 1 tbsp. low-fat Italian dressing

- 1 cup carrots, julienned

Instructions:

1. Put the dressing and tuna in a bowl and mix well.

2. Arrange half of the mixture on one of the tortillas. Add half the amount of each vegetable and wrap.

3. Do the same to the remaining tortilla.

Sun Crust Turkey Cuts

Ingredients:

- 2 turkey breasts, cut into 1/4-inch thick slices

- 1-1/2 cups sunflower seeds

- 1/4 tsp. ground cumin

- 2 tbsp. chopped parsley

- 1/4 tsp. paprika

- 1/4 tsp. cayenne pepper

- 1/4 tsp. black pepper

- 1/3 cup whole wheat flour

- 3 egg whites

Instructions:

1. Preheat the oven to around 395 °F.

2. Mix the parsley, paprika, cumin, cayenne, sunflower seeds, and pepper in a processor.

3. Prepare the whites and flour in a separate container each.

4. Coat each breast part with the mixtures separately. Start with the flour mixture, followed by the whites, and then the processed mixture.

5. After coating all the breasts, prepare the pan.

6. Bake the breasts for approximately 12 minutes in the oven.

7. Flip each side and resume baking for another 12 minutes.

8. Serve hot.

Tomato and Turkey Panini

Ingredients:

- 3 tbsp. fat-reduced mayonnaise

- 1 tsp. lemon juice

- 2 tbsp. plain, non-fat yogurt

- freshly ground pepper

- 2 tbsp. shredded parmesan cheese

- 8 pcs. sodium-reduced turkey, sliced thinly

- 2 tbsp. fresh basil, chopped finely

- 8 slices of tomato

- 2 tsp. canola oil

Instructions:

1. Combine parmesan, mayonnaise, yogurt, lemon juice, basil, and pepper in a bowl.

2. Spread 2 teaspoons of the mixture on each bread.

3. Divide tomato and turkey slices evenly among the four slices of bread. Top each with the remaining bread.

4. Heat a teaspoon of oil in a skillet over medium heat.

5. Place two panini in the pan. Place the skillet on top of the panini. Use the cans to weigh it down.

6. Cook the panini until they turn golden on one side, which may take about a couple of minutes.

7. Reduce the heat to low and fry the panini.

8. Repeat the same process on the other side. Cook the remaining Panini.

9. Serve and enjoy immediately.

Baked Turkey Wings

Ingredients:

- 4 pcs. or about 5 lbs. whole turkey wings

- 1 tbsp. olive oil

- salt

- pepper

- 1 tsp. paprika

Instructions:

1. Preheat the oven to 375°F.

2. Use foil to line a baking pan.

3. Remove the wing tips and fat. Separate from the drumette.

4. Place on the rack and drizzle with olive oil.

5. Season with pepper and salt.

6. Roast turkey wings until cooked.

7. Sprinkle paprika over the wings upon serving.

Crock Pot Chicken Soup

Ingredients:

- 6 pcs. chicken legs, skinless
- 2 carrots, chopped
- 1 onion, sliced
- 5 cloves garlic, minced
- 1 tbsp. olive oil
- 5-1/2 cups of water
- dried herbs or Italian seasoning
- salt
- pepper

Instructions:

1. Put carrots, onion, and garlic in the slow cooker. Add salt, pepper, and dried herbs, to taste. Add olive oil.

2. Crush the bones of the chicken, breaking the cartilage. Arrange on top of the vegetables in the pot.

3. Add water.

4. Set the slow cooker to low. Cook for 8-10 hours.

5. Add more seasoning if desired. Serve hot.

Salmon Soup

Ingredients:

- 1-3/4 cup coconut milk

- 2 tsp. dried thyme leaves

- 4 leeks, trimmed and sliced into crescents

- 6 cups seafood stock or chicken broth

- salt, for seasoning

- 3 cloves garlic, minced

- 1 lb. salmon, cut into bite-sized pieces

- 2 tbsp. avocado oil

Instructions:

1. Place avocado oil in a large saucepan or Dutch oven at low-medium heat. Add garlic and leeks.

2. Cook vegetables until slightly softened.

3. Pour in chicken or fish stock. Add in thyme and allow the mixture to simmer for approximately 15 minutes.

4. Season with salt to taste.

5. Add both coconut milk and salmon.

6. Bring the mixture up to a gentle simmer.

7. Cook until the fish is tender and opaque, then serve while hot.

__Barley and Chicken Soup__

Ingredients:

- 4 cups vegetable broth
- 4 cups chicken broth
- 2-1/2 lb. chicken breast, cubed, bone and skin removed
- 2 cups butternut squash, peeled and cubed
- 2 cups yellow summer squash
- 2 cups cubed zucchini squash
- 1 cup white onion, diced
- 1 cup broccoli florets
- 8 oz. fresh mushrooms, chopped
- 1 cup barley
- 2 cups water
- 1 tbsp. garlic, minced
- 1 whole bay leaf
- 1/4 tsp. sea salt
- 1/4 tsp. ground black pepper

Instructions:

1. Pour the water, vegetable broth, and chicken broth in a large pot.

2. Add the chicken cubes, onion, garlic, bay leaf, salt, and black pepper.

3. Using medium-high heat, bring the contents of the pot to a boil.

4. Reduce the heat to low. Simmer for an hour.

5. Add the barley, broccoli, butternut squash, yellow summer squash, zucchini, and mushrooms into the pot.

6. Bring back to a boil.

7. Lower it to a simmer for about 60 to 120 minutes, or until vegetables have achieved your desired texture.

8. Transfer into a serving bowl immediately.

Apple and Onion Soup

Ingredients:

- 3 organic apples, diced
- 2 medium yellow onions, sliced
- 6 cups vegetable broth
- 1 small leek, chopped
- 1 tbsp. avocado oil
- 1/2 tbsp. fresh rosemary, chopped
- 1/2 tbsp. fresh thyme

Instructions:

1. Place the saucepan over medium heat.

2. Pour the avocado oil into the saucepan.

3. Add the onion slices. Sauté until the color has turned golden.

4. Pour in the vegetable broth.

5. Bring to a boil over medium heat.

6. Add the diced apples.

7. Reduce the heat to the medium-low setting.

8. Simmer for 10 minutes.

9. Serve immediately.

Conclusion

Tailbone pain or coccydynia is a serious condition that can greatly affect a patient's daily routine. The pain can become unbearable depending on how grave the injury is. To attempt to avoid making the condition worse, there are other things recommended and suggested for you to do to manage the pain and the injury.

Treatments for tailbone pain are available, depending on what exactly you need for your injury, which will be determined by your doctor. However, this does not mean there is nothing you can do to manage the discomfort of having tailbone pain. Learning how to manage the condition in the comforts of your own home will not only make your daily routine much more bearable to do, but you can also help your tailbone and the muscles surrounding it be more capable of protecting your coccyx.

Switching to healthy diets, doing stretching and strengthening exercises, and following after-care routines religiously will definitely help. You may recognize the difference before and after doing all these things to manage the pain. While it may not entirely cure the tailbone injury, allowing it to heal by not adding more stress and helping it be stronger will be extremely beneficial to you in the long run.

References

5 best home remedies to treat tailbone pain. (2014, December 10). STYLECRAZE. https://www.stylecraze.com/articles/effective-home-rem edies-to-treat-tailbone-pain/.

Coccyx injections. (n.d.). NOVA Interventional Pain and Spine. Retrieved November 20, 2022, from https://www.novainterventionalpain.com/services/coccy x-injections/.

MD, R. S. (n.d.). Coccygectomy surgery for coccydynia(Tailbone pain). Spine-Health. Retrieved November 20, 2022, from https://www.spine-health.com/conditions/lower-back-pa in/coccygectomy-surgery-coccydynia-tailbone-pain.

MD, R. S. (n.d.). Treatment for coccydynia(Tailbone pain). Spine-Health. Retrieved November 20, 2022, from https://www.spine-health.com/conditions/lower-back-pa in/treatment-coccydynia-tailbone-pain.

Ogur, H. U., Seyfettinoğlu, F., Tuhanioğlu, Ü., Cicek, H., & Zohre, S. (2017). An evaluation of two different methods of coccygectomy in patients with traumatic coccydynia. Journal of Pain Research, 10, 881–886. https://doi.org/10.2147/JPR.S129198.

Physiotherapy, C. B. (n.d.). What is tailbone pain and how physiotherapy can help! | blog by cb physiotherapy, active healing for pain free life. Cbphysiotherapy. Retrieved November 20, 2022, from

https://cbphysiotherapy.in/blog/what-is-tailbone-pain-and-how-physiotherapy-can-help.

sovetplus.com. (n.d.). 5 ways to get rid of tailbone pain. Useful Home Tips | Sovetplus.Com. Retrieved November 20, 2022, from https://sovetplus.com/en/health/health-and-medicine/5-ways-to-get-rid-of-tailbone-pain

Tailbone (Coccyx) pain. (2017, October 23). NHS.UK. https://www.nhs.uk/conditions/tailbone-coccyx-pain/.

Tailbone pain (Coccydynia): Causes, treatment & pain relief. (n.d.). Cleveland Clinic. Retrieved November 20, 2022, from https://my.clevelandclinic.org/health/diseases/10436-coccydynia-tailbone-pain.

Tailbone pain: Overview, causes, and treatment. (2015, January 22). Healthline. https://www.healthline.com/health/back-pain/tailbone-pain.

Vertebral column—An overview | sciencedirect topics. (n.d.). Retrieved November 20, 2022, from https://www.sciencedirect.com/topics/neuroscience/vertebral-column.

Printed in Great Britain
by Amazon